AF485820

Copyright © 2021

All rights reserved. No part of this publication maybe reproduced, distributed, or transmitted in any form or by any means, including photocopying, recording, or other electronic or mechanical methods, without the prior written permission of the publisher, except in the case of brief quotations embodied in critical reviews and certain other noncommercial uses permitted by copyright law.

Contents

Okinawa Diet

Okinawa is a 466 square mile island in the Pacific Ocean, 400 miles south of Japan. The current population is around 1.3 million people and up until recently, the average life expectancy of Okinawa residents was 81.2 years, which was the longest in the world. The majority of Okinawans reside on Okinawa Island, but the entire region is known as a "blue zone," a place where people not only live longer but also healthier, with fewer age-related diseases.

Since 1975, scientists have been researching the centenarians of Okinawa to understand the reasons behind their long lifespans. Many have observed that the traditional Okinawa diet plays a significant role in Okinawan health and longevity. What the Okinawa diet plan attempts to do is mimic the island's traditional foods and eating habits, before it transitioned to the Westernized diet late last century. The regional diet consists of mostly vegetables and legumes, especially soy. It's low in calories and fat, high in fiber, and includes complex carbohydrates.

"Features such as the low levels of saturated fat, high antioxidant intake, and low glycemic load are likely contributing to a decreased risk for cardiovascular disease, some cancers, and other chronic diseases," one study reported.

Salient features of Okinawa diet

1. Calorie restricted diet: The diet of the Okinawan people is 20% lesser in calories than an average Japanese consumes. Their food is consistently averaging no more than one calorie

per gram, and the average Okinawan has a BMI (Body Mass Index) of 20. Many research studies firmly suggest the human body receives more harmful free radicals from food than they through external agents like bacteria, viruses, chemicals, etc.

Calorie restriction, therefore, is thought to improve health and slow the aging process in some animal models like rodents by limiting their dietary energy intake below the daily average needs.

2. Antioxidant-rich diet: Okinawa diet composes mainly green/orange/yellow (GOY) vegetables, fruits, roots, and tubers. These foods are rich sources of antioxidant vitamins like vitamin-C, vitamin-A, and flavonoid polyphenolic

compounds like ß-carotenes, lutein, xanthins, and minerals like calcium, iron, potassium, and zinc.

3. Low in fat and sugar: The Okinawa diet is low in fat, has only 25% of the sugar and 75% of the cereals of the average dietary intake of a Japanese. Limiting fat and sugar in the diet can help prevent coronary heart diseases and stroke risk.

4. Vegetarian and seafood rich: The islander's traditional diet includes a relatively small amount of fish and somewhat more in the form of soy, low-calorie vegetables like bitter melon, and other legumes. Almost no meat, eggs, or dairy products are consumed. Fish provides omega-3 essential fatty acids like alpha-linolenic acid

(ALA), eicosapentaenoic acid (EPA), and docosahexaenoic acid (DHA). Besides being an excellent source of protein, soy (in the form of tofu), contains health benefiting compounds like soluble dietary fiber, tannin antioxidants, and plant sterols. Altogether, these phytonutrients offer protection against heart diseases, stroke, colon, and prostate cancers.

The advocates of Okinawa diet divide food items into four categories based on their caloric density, as follows:

• The "featherweight" foods: Food groups that provide less than or equal to 0.8 calories per gram belong to this category. Citrus fruits like orange, low-calorie vegetables like spinach, cucumber, etc. One can eat many servings per day without any reservations.

• The "lightweight" foods: Food items with a calorific density of 0.8 to 1.5 per gram fall in this category. Certain fruits like banana and vegetables like potato are examples in this category. One should consume these in moderation.

• The "middleweight" foods: Food group having a caloric density from 1.5 to 3.0 calories per gram, such as cereals like wheat, legume products, and lean meat included under this category. It advised that one should eat only while carefully monitoring the portion size.

• The "heavyweight" foods: Food items which provide 3 to 9 calories per gram (300 to 900 calories per 100 g) belong in this category. Many oils and fats, nuts, oil seeds and red meat fall in this category, which one should eat only sparingly.

Okinawa diet is simple and close to nature. It composes mainly of green/orange/yellow (GOY) vegetables, fruits, roots, and tubers and simple seafood. On an average, each Okinawan consumes no more than one calorie per gram of food and median BMI (Body Mass Index) is 20.

How Does the Okinawa Diet Lead to Longevity?

So how, precisely, may this plant-forward diet contribute to blowing out 100 candles on the proverbial birthday cake? "One of the reasons the Okinawa diet may help with longevity is the high antioxidant content. Plant-based foods, including the sweet potato, are high in antioxidants and protect against disease to extend life," shares Jinan Banna, Ph.D., RD, referencing this 2016 study.

"In addition, [the] caloric restriction also likely contributes to longevity in Okinawa, though the biological basis for this is still being researched," Banna also notes, pointing to this 2014 study on caloric restriction and healthy aging in Okinawa.

What Can You Eat?

Typical foods in the Okinawa diet include a variety of sweet potatoes, soy, bitter melon (goya), shiitake mushrooms, burdock, jasmine tea, seaweed, and an array of herbs and spices like moringa and turmeric.

Most of the carbohydrates in the Okinawa diet come from vegetables, with a smaller amount from fruits, grains, or seeds. Abundant in the region is the acerola fruit (which is packed with vitamin C and antioxidants) and the Okinawa lime known as shikwasa, a citrus fruit rich in polyphenols and antioxidants. While these fruits may be hard to come by in the U.S., Americans can look to the anti-aging benefits of vitamin C and antioxidants for longevity.

The diet does not contain added sugars or refined sweets, with the exception of uji, Okinawan sugarcane, which is boiled down to make brown sugar and is also used to encourage healthy digestion. Okinawans eat a little pork and a minimal amount of dairy. Fish is consumed in moderation, and alcohol consumption is limited to an occasional drink.

• Eat more vegetables. Fill your plate with plenty of deep green or brightly colored veggies.

• Choose soy and soy foods. Try adding tofu to a stir-fry or switch from dairy milk to soy milk. Or experiment with natto, a fermented soybean dish.

• Add mushrooms to your meals. Try different varieties like shiitake, oyster, and king trumpet mushrooms. They can take the place of meat as the focus of a meal.

What to Eat

• Dark leafy vegetables

- Sweet potatoes (orange, yellow, and purple)

- Seaweed

- Fish (in small amounts)

- Bitter melon (goya)

- Legumes, especially soybeans

- Burdock root

- Shiitake mushrooms

- Herbs and spices

- Dashi (soup stock)

What Not to Eat

- Meat (except occasionally)

- Dairy products (except occasionally)

- Grains (white rice and noodles on occasion)

• Sugar

Okinawa Diet Food Groups

• According to an April 2014 study in the Mechanisms of Ageing and Development journal and a July 2016 study in the journal Age and Ageing, Okinawa nutrition was primarily plant-based, with root vegetables as the primary components.

• If you want to try a traditional Okinawa diet, the study in Mechanisms of Ageing and Development says that you'll end up consuming around 58 percent of your calories from vegetables. The staple of the Okinawa diet is the sweet potato, but other root vegetables and leafy greens were also commonly consumed.

- The second biggest category included in the Okinawa diet comes from grains. Around 33 percent of calories come from whole grains. Rice did not grow well on Okinawa, but the traditional diet did feature other grains, like millet.

- Legumes are the third largest component of the Okinawa diet. However, they only make up 5 percent of the total calories consumed if you follow the diet. The remaining dietary calories are from fatty foods, sugary foods and animal products. Two percent of calories come from oils, while 1 percent of calories come from fish and other seafood products. Less than 1 percent of calories come from nuts and seeds, sugars, meat products, eggs, dairy and fruit.

- You should be aware that there is some disagreement regarding the dietary proportions of the Okinawa diet. Older studies, like the Annals of the New York Academy of Sciences study, state that around 74 percent of calories came from vegetables, while 19 percent of calories came from grains. But ultimately, this difference is minor.

Both studies agree that 91 to 93 percent of daily calories came from vegetables and whole grains, with animal and seafood products making up just 2 to 3 percent of daily calories.

Okinawa food list

Depending on the source you reference, the list of foods found in the diet will include the following items. However many were in minuscule quantities and not eaten on a daily basis.

Grains and grain products

o brown rice

o white rice

o soba noodles

o rice noodles

o seitan – vital wheat gluten

Soba is actually the Japanese word for buckwheat, which despite its name, is actually in the same family as rhubarb and is not related to wheat. Traditional soba noodles are gluten free, however the pre-made varieties you can buy at the grocery store today are usually a mix of 50% buckwheat and 50% wheat, because diluting the ingredient with wheat makes it cheaper to produce. With the exception of seitan (which not all sources even reference), the Okinawa diet consists largely of gluten free ingredients.

Vegetables

o purple sweet potatoes

o goya/bitter melon – also known as the balsam-pear

o seaweed – primarily kombu and mozuku

o taro root

o hechima/luffa – a tropical and subtropical cucumber species

o shikwasa – also called the shequasar, flat lemon, and Taiwan tangerine

o okra

o Okinawan carrots – long and light yellow in color

o garlic

o tomato

o handama – a leafy vegetable with green and purple leaves

o shima rakkyo – similar to a shallot

o onions

o salad leaves

Legumes

o tofu

o miso

o soy sauce – only minuscule amounts, as the traditional diet is very low sodium

Soy foods in particular are very important and consumed on a daily basis. The authors of The Okinawa Diet Plan have stated that the islanders ate more tofu than any other culture in the world, even more than mainland Japan, the Chinese, and other Asian countries.

bottle of shiikwasaa juice (10% shiikwasaa) which is sold on the Okinawan islands, photo by Artuu at English Wikipedia

Fruits

o bogor pineapple – also known as the snack pineapple, you can pick apart the fruit by hand without the need for a knife

o shiikwaasaa – also called a flat lemon, it's a popular citrus fruit which contains nobiletin, a flavanoid which has recently been studied for anti-inflammatory and anti-cancer properties in vitro as well as animal studies

o mangos

o papaya

o passion fruit

o guavas

o acerola cherry – one of the richest sources of vitamin C

Meats, fish, and seafood

o fish – gurukun, tuna, and malabar grouper have gained popularity, however traditional Okinawa cooking used very tiny amounts of fish in their recipes (less than a half serving per day) o beef – moderate consumption of beef is a

newer trend

o goat – a less common form of meat that

Okinawans would eat

Condiments

o koregusu – a distilled liquor with chili peppers

in the bottle, typically only a few drops would be

used to add a hint of flavor to dumpling sauce,

noodles, and other recipes

o soy sauce – only small amounts

o sea salt – only small amounts

Okinawa Diet Calorie Consumption

- The Okinawa diet is well known for being a low-calorie, carbohydrate-rich diet. However, the number of calories you should consume while following the Okinawa diet is often misreported. Calorie intake should be based on multiple factors, including your gender, body size and activity level.

- According to an October 2007 study in the Annals of the New York Academy of Sciences___, the Okinawan people in the mid-20th century ate very few calories compared to people today. In fact, the average Okinawan had a negative energy balance of about 218 calories per day.

- If you were to take factors like body size into account, the equivalent would be the consumption of around 1,785 calories per day instead of the standard 2,000-calorie diet. However, on any given day, a person's total food consumption could range between 1,605 total calories and 2,012 total calories.

• If you're planning to follow an Okinawa diet plan, you should be conscious of your calorie consumption. According to Harvard Health Publishing, women should not consume less than 1,200 calories per day, while men should not consume less than 1,500 calories on a daily basis.

•

Traditional Okinawan Breakfasts

• Okinawan breakfast, lunch and dinner were all served with jasmine tea. All meals were also likely to feature the sweet potato in some shape or form.

• The study in the Mechanisms of Ageing and Development journal states that about 965 grams of vegetables were consumed each day. Because the average medium-sized sweet potato is 251 calories, this means that around three sweet potatoes were consumed per day. The remaining 200-odd calories likely came from fiber-rich vegetables like bitter melon, daikon radish, okra, carrots, pumpkin, cabbage, bamboo shoots and sea vegetables.

• Japanese breakfasts often feature soybeans, miso soup, and eggs. A typical Okinawa breakfast recipe was likely grain-based, featuring foods like brown rice and fermented soybeans (known as natto). Congee a type of porridge commonly consumed in Asia, may have also been served with vegetables or soy products.

- Miso soup is also a popular breakfast dish. While the Okinawa diet is heavily plant-based, it still involves meat and seafood. All parts of an animal were consumed — even things like pig ears and feet. This means that Okinawa vegan recipes weren't actually that common.

- Even when actual meat or offal weren't available, fish and meat broths were produced from bones. These broths were mixed with miso paste to produce the miso soup. This version of miso soup also included tofu, fish, vegetables, resulting in a product that's very different from the traditional mainland Japanese version of this soup.

Traditional Okinawan Lunch and Dinner

• Creating a fish, chicken stock, skimming off the fat and using the broth to make stews or stir-fries is also an easy way to produce a flavorful lunch or dinner. This is known as the champuru style of cooking. Stir-fries of bitter melon, cabbage and bamboo would often be served alongside small amounts of fish, pork, tofu or the occasional egg.

• There are two other styles of cooking common in Okinawa. The nbushi style of cooking mixes miso (a soybean paste) with vegetables like daikon radish, okra, carrots and pumpkin to produce stews and soups. These vegetables contain a lot of water, so they essentially release liquid as they cook, resulting in a rich, flavorful dish.

• Finally, the irichi style of cooking simmers or stir-fries vegetables or fruits like papaya on their own. No actual legumes, meat or fish were integrated, but sometimes fat that had been skimmed off of chicken broths was used instead of a vegetable or seed oil.

• Alongside these vegetable dishes, you also would find side dishes of mugwort, marinated seaweed or sauteed greens from the sweet potato plant. Dinner would often end with small amounts of fruit served as a dessert. Brandy made from the millet grain was also consumed on special occasions.

Health Benefits

Lower Risk for Chronic Disease

A low-fat, low-calorie, and high-fiber diet rich in antioxidants is quite possibly a main contributing factor to the excellent health of the Okinawan people. The Okinawa diet could also help you lose weight and promote healthy weight management, which is essential for avoiding chronic diseases like cardiovascular disease, diabetes, and some forms of cancer.

May Reduce Inflammation

The anti-inflammatory properties of the Okinawa diet can help reduce the risk of those chronic diseases for a number of reasons. The diet is:

• Low fat (especially saturated fat), but still high in omega-3 fatty acids. At least some forms of saturated fats can increase inflammation and omega-3's help reduce inflammation.

• Low in refined carbohydrates (like sugar), so it doesn't have a big impact on your blood sugar levels. Blood sugar spikes can contribute to a pro-inflammatory state in your body that increases the risk of chronic disease and inflammation.

• High in vitamins C, E, and A and phytochemicals. These nutrients work as antioxidants to protect your cells from free radical damage (things like smoke, pollution, rancid fats and oils, and so on). These nutrients may also help to reduce inflammation.

Health Risks

Very Restrictive

Though there are no common health risks associated with the Okinawa diet, restricting food groups like complex carbs, dairy, and animal products could result in nutrient deficiencies and even an unhealthy obsession with clean eating.

The Okinawa diet is very low in red meat, eggs, and poultry, but you may still be able to get enough protein from soy, fish, and the occasional pork. You may also be able to get enough nutrition without whole grains and dairy, but it can be difficult to follow a diet that's this restrictive for the long term.

High in Sodium

If you're on a salt-restricted diet, speak to your doctor before adding in some of the sodium-rich foods on this diet like miso, salted fish, or soy sauce (even reduced-sodium soy sauce is high in sodium). It's possible the abundance of fruits and vegetables also included in the diet that are high in potassium and calcium could counteract the sodium,[11] but it's better not to risk it.

Sample Meal Plan

The Okinawa diet limits grains like white rice and noodles and instead emphasizes plenty of vegetables and legumes, especially sweet potatoes. Since it may not seem ideal to eat a sweet potato at every meal, you can incorporate other foods like edamame, miso soup, sauteed greens, and of course, plenty of seaweed. Served on top of noodles, in salads and stir-fries, and with vegetables, seaweed is a versatile sea vegetable that can add more flavor to your dishes on the Okinawa diet.

The following three-day meal plan is inspired by the Okinawa diet but is not all-inclusive. If you choose to follow an Okinawan-inspired diet, there may be other meals that better suit your tastes and preferences. You can accompany these meals with water, jasmine tea, or the occasional low-alcohol beverage with dinner.

Day 1

- Breakfast: 1 cup of miso soup with dashi and kombu; tofu and mushroom "scramble" (no eggs)

- Lunch: Baked sweet potato (orange, yellow, or purple); 1/2 cup white rice; 1/2 cup edamame

- Dinner: 4-ounce portion oven-baked salmon; 1/2 cup bok choy and oyster mushroom stir-fry

Day 2

- Breakfast: Kale and sweet potato hash (with an optional fried egg)

- Lunch: 1 cup of seaweed salad with pickled burdock root; 1 onigiri rice triangle; 1/2 cup natto

- Dinner: 1 cup broccoli stir-fry (omit the sugar); 1/2 cup pan-seared tofu or a 4-ounce serving of simmered pork belly

Day 3

- Breakfast: 1 cup of miso soup with dashi and hijiki; 1 soft-boiled egg

- Lunch: 1 cup kinpira gobo (burdock root and carrot stir-fry); 1/2 cup of roasted purple sweet potatoes

Dinner: 1 1/4 cup serving of peanut noodles with tofu and vegetables

OKINAWA DIET RECIPES

Trying a okinawa-friendly recipes is a great way to explore new flavors and find new favorite dishes while looking after your health. In this part are nourishing okinawa diet recipes for lifelong health.

Taco Rice

Preparation time

15 minutes

Ingredients

- 500 g Beef Mince OR Beef & Pork Mince

- 1 tablespoon Canola Oil

- 1 Onion

- 1 clove Garlic *finely chopped

- 2 tablespoons Tomato Paste

- 4 servings Freshly Cooked Rice

- 2-3 Lettuce Leaves *sliced

- 2 Tomatoes *cut into small pieces

- 1 Avocado *cut into small pieces

- Shredded Cheddar Cheese

Taco Salsa

1. 2 teaspoons Ground Cumin

2. 2 teaspoons Ground Coriander

3. 1 teaspoon Garlic Powder

4. 1 teaspoon Paprika

5. 1/8 teaspoon Cayenne Pepper *OR more

6. 1 teaspoon Salt

Instructions

1. Heat Oil in a large frying pan over medium-high heat, cook Onion and Garlic for a few minutes, add Beef Mince and cook until Beef changes colour.

2. Add the spices mix and Tomato Paste, and stir-fry for a few minutes.

3. Place Freshly Cooked Rice on a plate, cover with the Beef mixture, then place Lettuce, Tomato, Avocado and shredded Cheese on top.

4. Drizzle with Taco Salsa and enjoy.

Goya Chanpuru

Preparation time

20 minutes

Ingredients

- 3 servings

- 1 goya

- 2 eggs

- 300 g sliced porks

- 1 handful bonito flakes

- 200 g tofu

- sesame oil

- salt and pepper

- soy sauce

Instructions

1. Slice the pork into 4cm, goya into 1cm, tofu into a bite size

2. Stir-fry the meat with one tsp of sesame oil

3. When the meat is well cooked, add the tofu and goya into the pan and fry together for 3 minutes

4. When the tofu start to get a little charcoal, season with salt and pepper.

5. Put the beaten egg and the bonito flakes into the pan, and pour soy sauce evenly from the edge of the pan.

Beef tacos rice

Preparation time

2 hours

Ingredients

- 3 cups rice

- 2 onions

- 4 garlic

- 8 tblspn of oil

- 4 maggi

- Pinch salt

- Spices

- 2 cups tomatoes and pepper paste

For the beef

- 3 large size of beef

- 4 pcs garlic

- 2 onions

- 1 scotch bonnet

- 1 maggi

- 1 tblspn of curry

- 1/2 cinnamon

- 1/2 cup water

- Pinch salt

Mayonnaise dressing

- 4 tblspn mayonnaise

- 3 garlic

- 1 tblspn red chilli flakes

- 1 scotch bonnet

- 1/2 tblspn black pepper

- 1/2 pepper paste

- Pinch salt

For the tortilla wraps (tacos)

- 1 cup flour

- 1/2 tblspn baking powder

- 3 tblpsn oil

- Pinch salt

- Water

Instructions

For the beef:

1. Add oil in a pot.

2. Add onions and garlic fry for a mnt.

3. Add ur spices and beef stir for 2 to 3 minutes.

4. Add Scotch bonnet and mix.

5. Add water and cover it to cook till soft

For the rice:

1. Add oil in a pot add the rice and stir till brown and transfer to a colander.

2. Add all the ingredients for the rice and cook for 2minuted and add the rice and water make sure it cover the top of the rice.

3. And cook until soft

For the tortilla:

1. Mix all the ingredients well.

2. Add water little at a time until u form a soft dough.

3. Knead the dough for 10 minutes,

4. cover it to rest for 5 minutes.

5. Roll it and bake in a pan 1½ mnt each side

For the mayonnaise:

1. Add all the ingredients and mix

The Tacos arrangement:

1. Add ur mayonnaise dressing.

2. flw by the beef and lastly the rice. cover the wrap egg wash the top.

3. Grease your pan with butter, add ur tacos add bake in low heat till golden brown and serve.

Handy Taco Rice

Preparation time

35 minutes

Ingredients

* 6 sheets of Rice paper (for summer rolls)

* Cooked rice made of 2cups rice

* 150 g ground beef

* 1 avocado

* 6 pieces mini tomato

* taco chips (tortilla chips)

* pizza cheese

seasonings

* 1/2 tea spoon chicken bouillon granule type

* 3 table spoons of ketchup

* 1/2 tea spoon cumin

Instructions

1. Roast ground beef in a Teflon pan and wipe off any excess fat.

2. Season the ground beef with seasonings.

3. Cook rice.

4. Slice the avocado.

5. Cut the cherry tomatoes in half.

6. Snack tortilla chips crush.

7. Soften the skin of summer rolls (rice paper) and place the rice in a long bale shape.

8. Make a hollow in the middle of the rice Put ground beef in the dent.

9. Put pizza cheese.

10. Finally, put taco chips (tortilla chips),

11. Place avocado in the top margin of the rice.

12. Put mini tomato.

13. Wrap everything in summer rolls. If you wrap it tightly, it will not collapse. You can use dried curry too.

Okinawan Carrots

Preparation time

15 minutes

INGREDIENTS

* 3 carrots medium to large sized

- 1 egg whisked

- 1 tsp soy sauce

- 1 tsp sesame oil

- 1 5 oz tuna canned tuna in oil – you will only use around 1/2 keep the rest to snack on!

- salt pinch of

- pepper pinch of

- water for cooking the carrots

- 1 green onion sliced for garnish

INSTRUCTIONS

1. Peel and julienne your carrots. The finer your carrots are julienned, the quicker they will cook!

2. Whisk one egg in a small bowl and leave it to the side.

3. Heat up a skillet to med-high.

4. Pour the oil from the tuna can into the skillet and heat up.

5. Once the oil is heated, add your carrots.

6. Stir fry for approximately 10 minutes or until softened.

7. Add a bit of water here and there to help the carrots cook. You don't want it watery though, so if you add water be sure to let the water burn off.

8. Once the carrots are soft and pliable, add the 1/2 can of tuna, breaking it up and stir.

9. Then add the soy sauce, sesame oil, and pinch of salt and pepper.

10. Lastly, add in your whisked egg, and continue stirring until the egg is cooked.

11. Remove and serve immediately, garnished with green onion!

Okinawa Tofu and Vegetables

Preparation time

15 minutes

Ingredients

- 1 cup sliced carrots

- 2 cups sliced onion white or yellow

- 1- 12-14 oz package firm tofu packed in water, drained and cut into 1/2 inch cubes

- 1-2 tablespoons olive oil

- 1 tablespoon butter optional but gives the dish good flavor

- salt and fresh ground pepper

- 2 tablespoons soy sauce

- 1-2 bunch of green onions white and green parts, sliced in 1" pieces, on diagonal

- sesame seeds for garnish optional

Instructions

1. Prepare all vegetables and tofu by washing, slicing and setting aside.

2. Place a medium to large size sauté or fry pan over medium to medium-high heat.

3. Add olive oil and butter to pan.

4. Heat until butter is melted.

5. Carefully add carrots and sliced yellow or white onion to pan.

6. Stir fry adding salt and pepper for about 3-4 minutes just until vegetables begin to soften.

7. Remove veggies from pan and set aside.

8. Add cut up tofu to pan and gently toss once or twice while cooking for about 3-4 minutes total.

9. Sprinkle soy sauce around and over tofu and add vegetables back to pan heat for another minute, do not toss at this point, or the tofu will fall apart.

10. Turn off heat.

11. Add sliced green onions to dish, sprinkle with sesame seeds (optional) and serve immediately with gohan (rice) and other sides if desired.

Okinawa Soba (Sōki Soba)

Preparation time

2 hours 30 minutes

Ingredients

- 400g/0.9lb egg noodles (note 1)

- 120g/5.3oz kamaboko or chikuwa , sliced to 7mm/¼" thick (note 2)

- 8 tbsp finely chopped shallots/scallions

- 4 tbsp beni shōga (note 3)

Sōki (makes more than 4 standard servings for Sōki Soba)

- 1kg/2.2lb pork rib strips (note 4)

- 30g/1.1oz ginger , sliced

Sōki Flavouring

- 65ml/2.2oz soy sauce

- 2 tbsp sugar

- 2 tbsp mirin

- 2 tbsp sake (note 5)

Soba Broth

- 1400 ml broth from boiling pork (note 6)

- 10g/0.4oz bonito flakes (note 7)

- 2 tsp salt

- 2 tsp soy sauce

- 2 tbsp mirin

- 1 tsp sake (note 5)

Instructions

1. Cut pork rib strip between the rib bones so that each piece gets meat with a bone (note 8).

2. Put the pork pieces in a pot and fill with water to fully cover the pork.

3. Bring it to a boil and cook for 5 minutes.

4. Drain and discard the fluid.

5. Rinse the pork pieces ensuring that scum is removed.

6. Remove the scums from the pot cleanly, return the pork to the pot and add ginger pieces.

7. Fill water to fully cover the pork pieces and bring it to a boil.

8. Reduce heat to low and simmer for 1.5 hours with a lid on, until the pork becomes very tender but not breaking easily.

9. Remove the pork pieces from the pot and keep the broth.

Making Simmered Sōki

1. Transfer the pork pieces to another large pot or a frying pan, preferably large enough to place the pork pieces in without overlapping.

2. Add the Sōki Flavouring ingredients to the pot/pan with the pork and bring it to a boil.

3. Reduce the heat to low and cook for about 5 minutes, turning the pork pieces over so that the flavour coats them.

4. Bring the heat to high and continue to cook until the sauce almost evaporates.

5. Turn the heat off.

Making Sōki Broth

1. Add bonito flakes to the broth and bring it to a boil.

2. Reduce the heat to simmer and cook for few minutes.

3. Put the broth through a sieve to remove ginger, bonito flakes and tiny pork bits (note 9).

4. Add the remaining Soba Broth ingredients and bring it to a boil.

5. Turn the heat off.

Making Sōki Soba

1. Boil water in a pot and cook noodles as per the instructions on the pack.

2. Drain water well and place noodles in each serving bowl.

3. Pour 350ml of the soba broth into each of the bowls, topped with the simmered sōki, kamoaboko/chiku

Easy and Authentic Okinawan Taco Rice

Preparation time

15 minutes

Ingredients

- 170 grams Mixed minced meat or minced beef

- 1/2 Onion

- 2 clove Garlic

- 1 tbsp Japanese-style Worcestershire sauce

- 2 tbsp Sweet chilli sauce

- 2 tbsp Ketchup

- 1 tsp Sugar

- 3 leaves Lettuce

- 1/2 Tomato

- 2 slice Easy melting cheese

- 2 Eggs

- 1 Nutmeg

Instructions

1. Mince the onion and garlic.

2. Heat some vegetable oil in a frying pan and fry until cooked.

3. Stir in the minced meat and fry until browned.

4. Sprinkle in the nutmeg and add the ingredients.

5. Mix all together.

6. Place a slice of cheese (without cutting it) over cooked rice.

7. Microwave at 500 W for 30 seconds to melt the cheese.

8. Top the melted cheese with the mixture from Step 2.

9. Place the shredded lettuce, diced tomatoes, and a fried egg on top.

10. Serve with ketchup to taste.

Tofu Vegetarian Taco Rice

Preparation time

17 minutes

Ingredients

- 150 grams Firm tofu

- 30 grams Kidney beans

- 50 grams Onion

- 1/2 Tomato (medium size)

- 1/2 clove Garlic

- 1 dash Salt and pepper

- 2 tsp Chili powder

- 1 tbsp Japanese Worcestershire-style Sauce

- 1 tbsp Ketchup

- 1 tsp Soy sauce

- 1/2 tbsp Vegetable oil

- 1 rice bowl Brown rice (or white rice)

- 5 slice Avocado

- 2 and 2 leaves Cherry tomatoes and lettuce

- 1 bunch Shredded cheese

Instructions

1. Wrap the tofu in two layers of paper towels and heat in the microwave for 2 minutes at 600 W.

2. Replace the paper towels.

3. Finely chop the onions, tomatoes, and garlic.

4. Heat the oil in a frying pan and stir-fry the garlic, onions, tofu, and tomatoes until the moisture evaporates.

5. Add the kidney beans.

6. Add the ingredients from above, then when the flavors are evenly distributed, add the soy sauce.

7. Pile the plate up with rice, then top with Step 4.

8. Add the avocado, tomatoes, cheese, and lettuce.

Healthy Veggie Taco Rice

Preparation time

30 minutes

Ingredients

- 1 block Koya tofu

- 1 small Carrot

- 1/2 Onion

- 1 Green pepper

- 3 leaves Lettuce

- 1 Baby leaves

- 5 Cherry tomatoes

- 1/2 Avocado

- 1/4 bunch Cilantro

- 1 tbsp Olive oil

- 50 ml Water

- 3 tbsp Ketchup

- 2 tbsp Japanese Worcestershire-style sauce

- 1 and 1/2 tablespoons Chili powder

- 2 tsp Soy sauce

- 1 Salt and pepper

- 2 servings Warm brown rice (or white rice)

- 1 Soy mayonnaise

- 1 Cheese (instead of soy mayonnaise)

- 1 Tortilla chips

Instructions

1. Soak the koya tofu in warm water.

2. Wash the vegetables and drain well before cutting.

3. Cut the lettuce into thick strips and the cherry tomatoes in half.

4. Avocado tends to change colour, so leave the cutting of that for later.

5. [Vegetarian Taco Meat] Drain any excess water off the tofu and blend in a food processor.

6. Finely chop the vegetables marked with .

7. Heat a frying pan and add some olive oil.

8. Stir fry the finely chopped vegetables marked with, then add the blended tofu and stir-fry together.

9. Once cooked, add the flavouring ingredients marked with and bring to the boil whilst continuing to stir fry.

10. Keep checking the taste of the meat, seasoning with a little salt and pepper to adjust. (I often add sauces, soy sauce, and chili here).

11. Now it's finally time to cut the avocado. If you have any, a few drops of lemon juice will help stop the avocado from changing colour.

12. Be careful not to add too much though, or the avocado may become too sour.

13. Put the cooked brown rice on a plate.

14. On top of that, add the vegetables marked with □, then the taco "meat", then the soy mayonnaise (or cheese).

15. Decorate with tortilla chips to finish.

Taco Meat for Taco Rice or Tacos

Preparation time

15 minutes

Ingredients

* 350 grams Ground beef (or a beef and pork blend)

* 1/2 Onion

* 2 clove Garlic

- 2 tbsp Japanese Worcestershire-style sauce

- 2 tbsp Ketchup

- 1 tbsp Sake

- 1 tbsp Chili powder

- 1 tsp Soy sauce

- 1 tsp Curry powder

- 1 Salt and pepper

- 1 Vegetable oil

Instructions

1. Mince the onion and garlic.

2. Heat vegetable oil in a frying pan and saute the garlic on low heat.

3. When the garlic becomes fragrant, add the meat and onion.

4. Season with salt and pepper and stir-fry while breaking apart the clumps.

5. When the meat begins to change color, mix in the ingredients.

6. Taste and if necessary, season with more salt and pepper to adjust the flavor.

Asian Somen Noodle Chanpuru with Fish Sauce

Preparation time

20 minutes

Ingredients

- 1 bundle Somen noodles

- 60 grams Pork offcuts or pork belly

- 2 bundles Komatsuna

- 1 tbsp Vegetable oil

- 1 clove Minced garlic

- 1 small piece Minced ginger

- 1/2 Takanotsume (sliced)

- 1 to 1 1/2 teaspoons Fish sauce

- 1 tsp Vinegar

- 2/3 tsp Shaoxing wine

- 1/2 tsp Salt

- 1/2 tsp Chicken soup stock powder

- 1 Pepper

- 1 Lemon juice

Instructions

1. Combine the seasonings.

2. Cut the komatsuna into 3 cm thickness, and cut the pork into suitable size.

3. Boil the somen noodles for a minute shorter than indicated on the package.

4. Rinse in cold running water and drain well.

5. Heat vegetable oil in a pan and saute the minced garlic, ginger and sliced red chile pepper, trying not to burn it.

6. When aromatic, add the pork to stir fry.

7. When the pork browns, add the somen noodles.

8. Pour the seasoning from Step 1 to the pan, add the chopped komatsuna, season with pepper.

9. Toss briskly and it's done.

Healthy Taco Rice

Preparation time

30 minutes

Ingredients

Meat sauce

• 200 grams Ground beef

- 1 large, chopped Onion

- 1/2 diced and blanched Cooked bamboo shoot in water

- 1 can. smush the tomatoes up will with your little hands. Canned tomatoes

- 1 Garlic

- 1 Whatever herbs and spices you have on hand

- 1 Bay leaf

- 1 dash Sake or wine

- 1 dash bit of each Ketchup, Japanese style Worcestershire sauce, soy sauce, sugar, salt, pepper

Salsa

- 1 as much (to taste), chop finely Tomatoes

- 1 as much (to taste), chop finely and put in a bowl of water Onion

- 1 swirl Olive oil

- 1 dash of each Lemon juice and parsley (optional)

- 1 dash of each Salt and pepper

- 1 Tabasco sauce

Vegetables of your choice

- 1 as much (to taste). roughly julienne. Lettuce, celery

Toppings

- 1 as much (to taste) Pizza cheese or cheese

Instructions

1. Let's make the meat sauce.

2. Stir fry the ground beef without oil.

3. Drain off any rendered fat.

4. Season with salt and coarsely ground black pepper, add the onion, bamboo shoot and a little sake, and stir fry.

5. Add whatever herbs and spices you have on hand, and as much as you like.

6. You can add red chili powder, oregano, paprika, nutmeg, black pepper, but the chili powder is a must.

7. Add a can of crushed tomatoes (juice and all) and one bay leaf.

8. Flavor with ketchup, Worcestershire sauce, soy sauce, sugar, salt and pepper. Adjust the quantity to your preference as you taste.

9. Even if you don't measure the ingredients, just taste as it cooks. When there's no liquid left in the pan, it's done.

10. Prepare the salsa.

11. Combine the salsa ingredients, adjust the seasoning with salt and pepper, and it's done.

12. Add Tabasco to taste.

13. Serve rice in a bowl, top with lots of vegetables, salsa, a generous portion of the meat sauce, cheese, and parsley.

14. Finished!! Add more Tabasco to taste.

Healthy Chanpuru Style Tofu Stir-Fry - Miso Is The Key

Preparation time

Ingredients

- 1/2 block （150 grams） Firm tofu

· 25 grams Kiriboshi daikon - dried shredded daikon radish

· 1/2 bunch Chinese garlic chives

· 30 grams Carrot

· 2 Shitake mushrooms

· 1 tbsp Miso

· 1 tbsp Sake

· 2 tsp Mirin

· 2 tbsp Japanese dashi stock

· 1 tsp Juice from grated ginger

· 1 tbsp Sesame oil

· 1 to 2 tablespoons Ground sesame seeds

Instructions

1. Wrap the tofu with kitchen paper towels and microwave for 1 minute. Leave to cool.

2. Soak the dried kiriboshi daikon radish in water to rehydrate and then cut into bite sized pieces.

3. Mix the ingredients marked together.

4. Cut the root end of the Chinese chives into 1cm-lengths, and the leafy part into 3cm-lengths.

5. Cut the carrot into thin rectanglular slices.

6. Slice the shitake mushrooms thinly.

7. Heat the sesame oil in a frying pan and add the carrot and dried daikon.

8. Stir fry over a medium to high heat.

9. Add the lower part of the Chinese chives and continue stir frying.

10. Add the leafy part of the Chinese chives and stir in.

11. Break up the tofu with your hands and add to the pan.

12. Stir gently so as not to break up the tofu pieces.

13. Stir in theingredients marked ◇ and turn off the heat.

14. Sprinkle on the sesame seeds and transfer to a serving dish - and you're done!

Taco Rice on Toast

Preparation time

Ingredients

· 1 Pizza type shredded cheese

· 1 1 cm cubed tomatoes

· 1 Ketchup flavored ground meat

Instructions

1. Place the ingredients on top of a piece of bread and toast!

2. I made this with the leftover taco rice after making some for my lunchbox.

3. You can use as much as you want on top of the bread!

Fashionable Lunch Taco Rice

Preparation time

12 minutes

Ingredients

- 100 grams Ground meat

- 1/2 Onion

- 1 pinch Garlic chips

- 1 dash Salt and pepper

- 1/4 a head Lettuce

- 1 Tomato

- 2 slice Easy melting cheese

- 2 Hot spring egg

- 2 tbsp Sweet chili sauce

- 1 tbsp Ketchup

- 1 tbsp Soy sauce

Instructions

1. Heat vegetable oil in a frying pan and sauté the garlic chips.

2. Add the onions and meat and stir-fry.

3. Once cooked through, use a paper towel to soak up excess oil.

4. Add the ingredients and combine.

5. Pile the rice on plates and top with the meat, then layer the strips of cheese on top. Microwave until the cheese melts, about 30 seconds at 550 W.

6. Shred the lettuce and chop the tomatoes into 1 cm chunks and add to the plate. Top with the hot spring eggand serve.

7. Drizzle on some Tabasco sauce on if you like.

Fish taco rice bowls

Preparation time

30 minutes

Ingredients

· 1 cup uncooked brown rice

· 1 3/4 cup water

· 1.25 lbs. mahi mahi, skin removed

· 1/4 teaspoon chipotle chili powder

· 1 teaspoon garlic powder

· 1 teaspoon smoked paprika

- 1/2 teaspoon salt

- 1/4 teaspoon ground black pepper

- 1 tablespoon canola oil

- 2 avocados, mash

- 2 tablespoons lime juice

- 2 cups purple cabbage, sliced

- 1 cup sliced jicama

- 1 cup diced roma tomatoes

- Picked Onions

Cilantro Lime Dressing:

- 1 tablespoon red onion

- 1 garlic clove

- 1 cup fresh cilantro

- 1/4 cup canola oil

- 2 tablespoons fresh lime juice

- 2 tablespoons red wine vinegar

- 1 tablespoon honey

- 2 teaspoons dijon mustard

- 1/4 teaspoon sea salt

- pinch ground cumin

Instructions

1. Add water and rice to a microwave safe bowl and cover.

2. Cook in microwave on HIGH for 10 minutes.

3. Let sit to cool and then fluff with a fork.

4. In a small bowl, add chipotle chili powder, garlic powder, smoked paprika, ½ teaspoon of salt, and ¼ teaspoon of black pepper.

5. Stir to mix.

6. Pat the fish dry and rub spice blend on both sides of the fish.

7. Heat large skillet to medium high heat.

8. Add 1 tablespoon of canola oil to the pan, then gently place prepared fish in pan.

9. Sear on both sides for 4-5 minutes.

10. Remove from pan and let rest.

11. To a food processor add red onion, garlic clove, fresh cilantro, ¼ cup of canola oil, lime

juice, red wine vinegar, honey, dijon mustard, ¼ teaspoon salt, and cumin.

12. Blend until smooth. Set aside.

13. In a small bowl, add mashed avocado and 2 tablespoons of lime juice.

14. Season with salt to taste.

15. Stir everything together.

16. Assemble the bowls: add ½ cup of rice, one filet of fish, a generous scoop of avocado mash, ½ cup purple cabbage, ¼ cup of sliced jicama, ¼ cup of diced tomato.

17. Drizzle with dressing mixture and serve!

Thai Style Rice Vermicelli Pad-Thai-Style Sōmen Chanpuru

Preparation time

20 minutes

Ingredients

· 2 bundles Sōmen noodles

· 1 handful Bean sprouts

· 1/2 bunch Chinese garlic chives

· 1/2 Japanese leek, minced

· 1 Your favorite vegetables (eg. cabbage, carrots, wood ear mushrooms, etc.)

· 1 Egg

· 2 rounds Takuan, chopped (optional)

· 1 dash Squid, shrimp, or pork (or sakura shrimp)

· 1/2 Aburaage or atsuage, choppped

· 10 Peanuts, chopped

· 3 tbsp Sweet chilli sauce

· 1 dash Soy sauce

· 1/2 clove Garlic

· 1/2 tsp Chicken stock granules

Instructions

1. Boil the sōmen noodles to a firm texture, drain, and rinse.

2. Cut the vegetables, squid, shrimp, or pork into bite-sized pieces. (Other than the bean sprouts or Chinese chives, any ingredients will do!)

3. Heat the oil in a frying pan, pour in the beaten egg, and scramble.

4. Transfer to a plate.

5. Add more oil to the frying pan and stir-fry the finely chopped leak and garlic until fragrant.

6. Add the squid, shrimp, pork, and aburaage or atsuage and stir-fry.

7. Turn the heat to high and add the vegetables and takuan.

8. Lightly stir-fry, then add 1/2 teaspoon of chicken soup stock granules dissolved into 1/4 cup of water.

9. Add the boiled sōmen noodles and quickly toss.

10. Season with soy sauce and sweet chili sauce.

11. Add the eggs from Step 2, transfer to serving plates, and top with the chopped peanuts to finish.

12. Drizzle with sweet chili sauce and top with lemon to taste.

Fajita & chicken tacos, rice

Preparation time

10 minutes

Ingredients

· 5 Corn tortillas

· 2 Fajita

· 1 Chicken breast

· 3/4 diced onion

· 1/2 green bell pepper

· Lemon and pepper

· Raw onion and cilantro

· 1/2 lime

Instructions

1. Starting with the fajitas only half way cooked then add the chicken breast while both chicken and fajita are cooking then you add the onion n the lemon pepper seasoning.

2. When done then you can just add it in your corn tortillas oh and add cilantro n raw onion or what ever you are pleased with....oh and you can add what ever salsa you like.

Stir-fried Goya (Goya Chanpuru)

Preparation time

15 minutes

Ingredients

· 1/2 (20 cm) goya (cut in half lengthwise, remove the seeds, cut into 3~5mm slices)

· 200 g firm tofu (drained and cut into bite sized pieces)

· 100~150 g pork or ham (cut into bite sized pieces)

· 1/2 sliced onion

· 1/4 carrot (cut into thin strips)

· 1~2 beaten eggs

Seasonings:

· 1 tbsp sake

· 1 tbsp soy sauce

· 1/2~1 tbsp oyster sauce

· 1 tbsp vegetables oil or olive oil for frying tofu

· 1 tbsp sesame oil

· dried bonito flakes for topping (optional)

· salt and pepper for seasoning

Instructions

1. Sprinkle salt on goya and rub, leave it for about 10 mins.

2. Wash with water and drain well.

3. Heat the oil (vegetable or olive oil) in a pan over medium heat, stir fry tofu until browned.

4. Remove tofu from the pan and set aside.

5. Heat the sesame oil in the same pan, add pork, onion, carrot, goya and stir fry for 1~2 mins(softened).

6. Put tofu back in the pan and then add seasonings and combine.

7. Pour the beaten egg over and stir quickly to mix.

8. Season with salt and pepper.

9. Top with dried bonito flakes (optional).

Taco Rice Casserole

Preparation time

1 hour 15 minutes

Ingredients

· 2 lb Ground Beef

· 1 Onion Chopped

· 1 Zucchini Shredded

· 2 C Corn

· 1 Can Black beans (drained)

· 1 Can Rotel

· 1 Package Taco seasoning

· Salt

· 4 C Cooked rice

· Handfuls shredded cheese

· 2 9x13 pans

Instructions

1. Brown beef. Add in Onion and zucchini and cook until soft.

2. Stir in taco seasoning.

3. Add corn, tomatoes and beans.

4. Spray 2 pans, spoon 2 C rice into the bottom of each pan.

5. Spoon the meat mixture over the rice.

6. Top with shredded cheese.

7. If you want to eat right away: bake covered at 350 for 25 min.

8. If freeze: let thaw overnight in fridge.

9. Bake at 350 for 45 min covered.

10. Then remove foil and cook until top is nice and brown.

OKINAWAN DOUGHNUTS

Preparation time

40 minutes

INGREDIENTS

- oil (for deep frying)

- 4 eggs

- 3/4 cup milk

- 3/4 teaspoon vanilla

- 4cups flour

- 2 cups sugar

- 3 1/2 tablespoons baking powder

- 1/4 teaspoon salt

Instructions

1. In a deep fryer or deep skillet, heat oil to 350 F or until hot.

2. In a large bowl, beat eggs, milk, and vanilla. Sift flour, sugar, baking powder and salt.

3. Add to egg mixture; stir until dry ingredients are moistened and dough is smooth.

4. Drop teaspoonfuls of dough into the hot oil; fry until golden brown and doughnuts rise to the surface.

5. Drain on paper towel lined plates and serve hot, but they are also good cooled down, you can buy them either way there on Okinawa!

Okinawa Sweet Potatoes

Preparation time

1 hour

Ingredients

· 4 pounds Okinawa (purple) sweet potatoes or white sweet potatoes, scrubbed

· 2 limes

· 1/4 cup butter

· Hawaiian red clay salt or sea salt

Instructions

1. Bring a large pot of water to a boil over high heat.

2. Prick sweet potatoes with a fork and boil until tender when pierced, 30 to 35 minutes.

3. Drain.

4. While potatoes are boiling, grate zest from limes and set aside; then squeeze juice from limes and set aside.

5. When potatoes are cool enough to handle, peel and slice into 1/2-in.-thick slices.

6. Arrange on a platter, cover with foil, and put in a 200° oven to keep warm.

7. Melt butter in a small saucepan over medium heat until foaming. Stir in zest and cook until fragrant, 1 minute.

8. Remove from heat and stir in lime juice.

9. Drizzle lime butter over potatoes and sprinkle with salt.

Okinawan salted shortbread

Preparation time

45 minutes

Ingredients

· 80 glard or vegetable shortening

· 60 gsoft dark brown sugar

· 150 gplain flour

· 1 tspsea salt flakes

Instructions

1. Heat your oven to 160°C.

2. In a medium saucepan, heat the lard and brown sugar together over low heat until liquid and combined.

3. Add the flour and mix to a soft dough.

4. Roll the dough between two sheets of baking paper to around 1cm thick and cut into 8cm x 3cm batons (using a crinkle cutter if possible).

5. Transfer the biscuits to a baking sheet and scatter with sea salt, lightly pressing it into the top of the biscuit.

6. Bake for around 25 minutes until firm.

7. Allow to cool before serving.

www.ingramcontent.com/pod-product-compliance
Lightning Source LLC
Chambersburg PA
CBHW071921120726
48001CB00005B/1815